Hacking Your Life in Western Society:

Living Techniques for Men in the Current Social Media Matrix

By MAURICE T. JOHNSON

Published 2019

ISBN: 9781695217720

Contents

PREFACE

Congratulations on being brave enough to take the first step on your journey to be the best version of yourself that you can be. We are all aware that men's spaces in westernized society are becoming increasingly more difficult to find and speak about pertinent topics when it comes to men's mental, physical and spiritual health. We are not allotted the same abundance of "safe spaces" as the opposite sex are.

In today's PC culture, men can be shamed, humiliated or can even lose their jobs just by speaking what is on their minds of their own free will as logical and thinking beings. Social conditioning currently makes it seem like men are less valuable than our female counterparts. The term "man up" is casually used in society to villainize men who believe in "traditional" family values such as patriarchy as misogynistic, homophobic or holding no accountability for their actions. Men are under constant attack when they refuse to follow society's norm.

Examples of such attacks are, slander by discriminatory news media who have had a history of prejudice and reporting false narratives for certain ethnicity groups in the United States. Similar entities have also resorted to the demonetization of popular channels by content creators on popular video sharing sites. General discussion by men on the topics of single motherhood, the women's sexual liberation, dating standards of millennial women, gender biasness in family court law or "men going their own way" could be considered too "controversial" resulting in whole channels being "shadow banned" a term used to describe a way that the media blocks a content creators content from the online community in such a way that it is not apparent that their content has been affected or even channels being terminated outright and without any notice, warning or explanation. These kind of actions continue to fuel social conditioning that creates a toxic environment that men have to tread cautiously in. We live in a time now where as a man living in a westernized country one small misstep could mean financial ruin or defamation of an individual's character and reputation.

This book is a collection of my personal thoughts through my own self journey of realization of one's true self and becoming the best version of myself that I can be. While I harbor no ill will towards any particular group of people or lifestyle choice know that I am a heterosexual and masculine male that believes in the right to live a comfortable and stress free life in any society. However, I feel that anyone can find and use the knowledge of this book to live more comfortable and meaningful lives while achieving their hopes and dreams.

I intend for this book to act as a guide to those that may be lost or starting over with their life while operating in the matrix of race and privilege in western society. Their time is up your time is now.

RULE 1: MOTIVATE YOURSELF

Motivate yourself by any means necessary. As a man living today in any westernized system it can seem to be an impossible task to be motivated about anything these days. Men face many social obstacles such as new age feminism, false #Metoo accusations, racism and profiling. Those perils are compounded by a constant barrage of negativity through the media and a "crabs in the barrel" mentality from so called "friends" and even family members. There are even economic factors such as racial wage gaps, gender and racial bias in the laws that govern the country. People have the ability to sue anyone for anything in this country with just an accusation and without any tangible evidence based on the ability to just pay. Given these factors it is not hard to feel depressed or ask yourself "why bother?"

Depression in men is a serious and under reported topic. Many men suffer in silence given the economic circumstances that they are raised in and negative environments that are forced to work under. Men are more likely to feel very tired or irritable when depressed. They may even lose interest in their passions, work or hobbies. They can become distant from significant people or friends in their life. Depression is usually seen as a sign of weakness in men. Men have become very proficient at hiding their feelings in plain sight. With no support groups these men suffer in silence. Male depression was brought to mainstream last year with the death of the beloved, Anthony Bourdain yet, past media interviews only hinted at depression attributing to his death.

I had a childhood friend that committed suicide over a girl. In my own personal life I have had to also deal with depression. I haven't been fortunate to have any support or support groups in the darkest moments of my life when I felt everything was hopeless and there was no light at the end of the tunnel. I made a personal choice not to succumb to those thoughts. Maybe it was my own ego of not letting the naysayers, exes or haters in my life win, but one day I woke up and made the effort to at least try. I recall telling myself if I failed then I just failed but at least I could say I tried and made an attempt. I knew I could look myself in the mirror and rest easily at night knowing that my attempt was for me and my well-being alone.

Remember suicide is NEVER the answer.

If you don't have a support group and you can't drag yourself out your bed to do whatever you want to set your mind too then who will? It has been quoted that,

"We are our own worst enemy."

These words could not be any truer. The biggest enemy you will have to deal with is yourself. This will be the hardest part in starting your journey and it is essential that you overcome this task. Whenever you venture into uncharted territory there is going to be doubt especially if you are serious and committed to making real change in your life.

You will have to train yourself to look past the social obstacles mentioned earlier and dedicate your time into becoming the best version of yourself that you can be. I am not saying to "fake it till you make it" but I am saying to do just that. Is it really faking though when you are about trying to be the best version of yourself that you can be? A lot of what could be considered "fake it till you make it" is your true-self internalizing what you need to do in order to achieve your goals. Hell, professional wrestlers had play fights as kids and made fake championship belts. Many of them became successful athletes making millions of dollars as adults. When I was a kid I remember drawing video game maps in school and made up fake video games while in class. That translated into me having a successful video gaming career as a 3D Artist in my adulthood and my own video game company where I created my own original content.

Your happiness is your responsibility! It's is not your friends, family or even children's job to make you happy. If you aren't right and you can't take care of yourself, how are you going to be able to take care of anyone else? Do not let other people dictate how you feel! Those same people will continue their day without even a thought on how crappy a person that they were to you. Let karma come back around to collect. It is also not your responsibility to figure out how the universe will collect on to them. Just continue doing you and working towards your goals. Stop worrying about what people think. We only have one life and you need to be the director of your own movie!

RULE 2: THE POWER OF POSITIVITY

Surround yourself with the power of positivity. The power of positivity is such an underrated and misunderstood topic when it comes to masculine principles. Being positive doesn't mean that you have to go around grinning around all the time like an idiot. Personally I am not a person that naturally smiles a lot. It takes a lot to make me smile so if someone is privileged to get a smile from me then you know it's genuine.

What I mean by being positive is to put your mind in a positive high vibration to focus on your tasks at hand. The higher the vibrations that you give off and send to the universe the more successful you will be in succeeding in your tasks. Now I know some of you are reading this thinking what is this "Hocus Pocus" nonsense but let me explain with a practical example. I could be called what could be considered as a "gym rat." I value personal fitness and working out. I am not the biggest or the strongest person in the gym at first glance but I am in better shape and proportions than 90% of people at the moment. I like working out because I like the way it makes me feel and how my body looks.

Now when I go into the gym to work out on a hard day (every gym day for me is a hard day) I have to be in a certain positive mindset in order to push up the heavy weights I need in order to get stronger. Let's say today is a chest day and I am doing bench press. I dare not go under that bar with anything less than a high vibration and mindset or risk being crushed by a bunch of heavy weights. I usually train alone and do not use a spotter. I focus on my task at hand with the right mind frame and visualize success. Then my mind processes the information and my body reacts accordingly! This is not Hocus Pocus, these are things that we do as men every day and do not give a second thought to it. If we can apply this kind of thinking to a task such as going to the gym to achieve fitness goals then why can we not apply this type of thinking to every other aspect of our lives?

Ways to increase your positivity are to surround yourself with positive messages and quotes online. I know many of us use social media as a form of entertainment but we need to make that work for us as well on the journey. Reading positive material such as this book or similar material or making blog pages about positive happenings in your life will also help to raise your vibrations. I was inspired to see people making Instagram and Flickr pages with nothing but positive quotes and pictures and that media influenced me on how I handle my own social media following and posts currently.

So many people view and use the internet and social media in a negative way. Rather it be gossiping or bullying it is usually not constructive or solution-oriented. Even viewing pages of friends and family living their best perceived lives can make put men in a depressed state. You get caught up in the perception of people living their best life and passing you up while you may be struggling or living check to check. However we don't know their reality is behind the scenes in the real world.

"Remember, people only show their best life on social media."

Talking to positive people or studying successful people that you want to emulate is another way of being positive. When you talk to other successful and positive people there is a transfer of their energy on to you and the universe responds accordingly. Still think it is Hocus Pocus? Have you ever noticed that after talking with a negative person who may have had a bad day and then they want to vent to you how your day starts to be become just as bad? This is one of the reasons people tend to avoid negative people. When asked about a winner's mindset, rapper Notorious Big said,

"Negativity brings failure.
We ain't trying to fail in this game, we are trying to succeed."

I am not saying that you cannot be a good friend and listen to others vent their feelings to you but you need to be aware that when you allow any type of negative energy into your essence that there is a transfer of energy from that person on to you. The universe is neutral it does not take sides. If this happens be sure to immediately work to re-center yourself into a positive mindset. I would suggest to try to avoid negativity completely.

Being negative also includes complaining something that I still struggle with to this day. A wise Sifu once mentioned to me not to put energy into things that I have no control over. Even in business you are told to surround yourself with like-minded individuals that are more successful then you. Learn to network regularly.

Listening to positivity through music is also another way of sending positive signals out to the universe in order to raise your vibrations to a higher level. It is a known fact that listening to music can improve your sleep, reduce stress and increase happiness. If it wasn't true that music doesn't have tangible effects on a person's physical state then people wouldn't be so concerned with listening to music while working out or when sitting behind a desk working.

The lyrics of music also have power as those lyrics are stored in your subconscious and brain. Music is memorable the same way we memorize other things. Our bodies and minds are in a constant influx of absorbing and processing the environments around them.

Have you ever thought about if the type of music that you listen to and if it actually compliments your life choices or beliefs? If the music you listen to is associated with positive memories it will most likely be used as a pick me up or confidence booster. However is the music you listen to is associate with negativity it may increase aggression or hyperactivity.

This is not necessarily bad but you should be aware of the psychological effects that you may experience while listening to the different types of music that you enjoy. You should always strive to put yourself and own well-being in the most positive light when working on your purpose. Music does change the way you feel and act.

RULE 3: VISUALIZATION

As men we are visual creatures. By visualizing things into your mind you are trying to will and manifest those things into reality.

I am huge fan of the creation of vision boards and writing down goals. I made a vision board of things that I would like to have in my life or material things that I would like have own one day. You can even start small. I challenge all of you to get postcard size piece of paper and use the internet to find some images of some things that you currently don't have or want in your life. It could be a luxury car, huge piles of money, a mansion, beautiful women etc. it doesn't matter. These are your own personal aspirations.

I even got my vision board cheaply laminated. You should place it somewhere where you will read or look at it every single day. This is the key. Even though you may haven't got to a point to where you can obtain those things yet, it should be the first thing you see in the morning or when you are working on your tasks to becoming the best version of yourself. Remember you are going to will these things into existence.

Another technique into visualizing your success is to actually go to similar locations you would like to live in one day. I like to drive through neighborhoods that contain luxury homes and visualize myself picking out the homes that would fit the lifestyle that I will eventually like to live one day. By doing this ever so often it helps to refocus me on my goals and gives me motivation to achieve the goals that I set for myself.

Additionally, this visualization sends positive signals out to the universe to manifest these things into existence. I have been fortunate enough because of my new lifestyle to have been privy to social gatherings in the very same type of spaces that I visualized about. My favorite car is the McLaren F1. It's one of the world's best and most expensive supercars. Recently, I continually been in areas and situations where I keep seeing this particular car in real life. This is the kind of affirmation that you are truly willing your aspirations into your own real life!

Writing down your goals keeps you accountable as well as focused on your tasks at hand. It is said that writing by hand also helps to improve your ability to remember things. Men have many unrealized goals and aspirations. Often it is easy to be overwhelmed by the sheer number of things that you may want to do or accomplish in your life! This is why it is so important to write things down.

Meditation is a great form of working on your visualization techniques. You can use mental imagery to become healthier or increase your confidence. It also reduces stress and helps to fight anxiety. Meditation helps to cultivate problem solving and enhances your self-awareness. A benefit of meditation is that you can use it anywhere at any time. If you are in an environment that does not allow for consistent alone or quiet time for yourself meditation is a great way of re-centering your vibrations and refocusing your efforts.

RULE 4: SELF- IMPROVEMENT

Being the best version of yourself always. This is a way of life and a lifestyle. Training is never over. Do not worry about other people. Also stop living in the past. It doesn't matter if it isn't 1996 anymore or whatever date you used to be successful in life. If you were able to be successful in one part of your lifetime then you never forget the talent in order to be successful again. It is hard wired into your very being.

Find the things you like to do that makes you happy and be about your purpose and then do those things a thousand fold. While you may haven't achieved your self-improvement goals at the moment, just the action of you making an attempt to work on yourself will build you the confidence in order to see the goals through till their completion. Additionally, self-improvement will give you the ability to navigate through negative situations or obstacles more easily. Whenever you are working on your purpose and being the best version of yourself that you can be, you will always keep forward momentum on your goals.

You should always strive to manifest your true self outwards into the world by your actions. It can even be something as simple as changing your wardrobe or perhaps adding more swagger into your attitude. Making a conscious effort into changing your body or even changing your hairstyle are other examples. By doing these types of things they will help you create a nonchalant and carefree attitude that will keep your vibration levels high so that you do not get derailed from your objectives. When you do this long enough it will become as natural as breathing. Your actions will manifest themselves onto other people and their perception on the way that they view you will start to change.

Have you ever had a situation where a woman rejected you in the past and then that person may see you years later when your social, economic or physical status has changed? Maybe you have been on your purpose and applying the techniques taught in this book into every aspect of your personal life. That very same woman will look at you differently maybe even becoming more receptive to you now. Now you have the power. You have the control. But you have had the control all along. What you needed was just focus, dedication and determination. You made a conscious effort to change yourself and you did it for no one but yourself and own well-being and happiness. That makes the victory even that much sweeter!

Men tend to stop trying to self-improve and evolve when their situation or their personal matters and environment overtake their purpose. You may have heard the horror stories from friends or family members that gave up their dreams and personal aspirations to live mediocre, unfulfilled and unhappy lives. They also tend to have a lot of self-regret and even self-loathing because they let other people that didn't care about them try to dictate their lives and their time. These people can also become low-key haters and may even be jealous of seeing you successful and try to hold you down! That is why it is so important for you to be able to block out the noise and continually self-improve. It is not your job to take other people with you on to your journey!

RULE 5: AVOIDING NEGATIVITY

This will be the second hardest rule that you will need to apply into your everyday life. This means to avoid all things negative and if something negative affects you trying to spin it into a positive. This also includes avoiding people who try to discredit you or by trying to bring you down to their level. This people could be called "blue pilled" people or people that have a "crab's in a barrel" mentality. These types of people will try to put doubt into you mind and may try to discourage you from achieving your goals. I strongly believe that:

> "You should avoid talking to people that cannot relate to your struggles."

I remember one day that I was in the gym on the bench press. I had already been in the gym doing super set's while benching up to 225lbs. for a few hours. Fatigued, I was on a drop set lowering the weight to 175lbs. I was on the my 8th or 9th repetition, when someone that I didn't know just jumped under my weight and started trying to spot me on their own. I immediately re-racked my own weight and told the individual that I had it under control and do not touch my bar when I am under that type of weight uninvited. People will try and project their own personal fears on to you. Especially, when you decide you want to change your life.

That particularly individual had been watching me in the gym earlier during my workout session and just happen to be lifting weights much lighter than what I was pushing. I am very observant and hyper focused on my goals when I am in the gym. This individual decided that he felt I needed some type of assistance even though his workout and weights were much lighter than mine.

These type of people may even try to low-key hate or "sneak diss" (disrespect) you. Putting a negative spin into at what first glance may seem like a genuine complement. Terms such as "you have more wins than losses" would be an example of a sneak diss someone may say to you. While they are acknowledging the fact that they see you are changing your life they subconsciously added a hint of negativity into their dialogue directed towards you. You must become hyper aware of these types of indicators. Sometimes negative people are unaware of themselves having this type of trait and it manifests itself outwardly subconsciously.

If one of your goals is to change your body you may even have people that will make comments such as "you aren't stronger than me" or "why would you eat or drink that" yet those people may be below the standards that you have set for yourself. These are examples of people that are projecting their own personal fears on to you.

These types of people are not your friend. They may even be family members. Do not be afraid to cut people off who are not adding value or on the same program as you out of your life! An important note about Rule #5 is to always try to have more positive aspects in your daily situations than negative. It is not going to happen overnight and this translates on how the universe responds to you on a daily basis. It is going to be different for everyone. This type of thought process has a direct correlation on how your body responds to your thoughts and external interactions with your environment. If you go into the gym with a negative attitude, the majority of the time your body tends to respond in an adverse way and your body won't be making any gains.

Negative people tend to become threatened by your success when they see you progressing and moving past in spite of them. They may even refuse to acknowledge your successes but they will still continue to pocket watch you. This is why Rule #1 is so important because you are not looking for anyone's validation when you are becoming the best version of yourself that you can be.

It is not your job or responsibility to change anyone else's perception of you. You will need to understand that no matter the amount of success that you achieve there will always be people that will just refuse to acknowledge it or will only perceive you a certain type of way even when you are obviously living your best life and have moved past them. It is best to not give any energy or thought to other people and just worry about what you are doing and living your best life!

Being negative tends to be unproductive and can emotionally and physically drain your essence throughout the day. It sends out bad signals to the universe and puts you in a lower vibration. You should use various techniques in order to help you to conquer it before it even starts.

One example is by changing your vernacular. Your subconscious mind can be very powerful. If you are an individual that constantly says, "I am sorry" too often you may send out signals to the universe that you are undermining your own value and self-worth. By changing the language and saying "I apologize" instead you are acknowledging your mistake in that moment only and moving on with your day.

You should also be actively thinking before you speak. Words are very powerful and once spoken you have spoken them you cannot take them back. If you take only a few moments before organizing your thoughts into language and you will be amazed how much more impactful and strategic you will be in your actions.

You need to own your behaviors unapologetically. By taking a moment to think before you speak it starts to train yourself into becoming more careful and meticulous in your actions. This will help you to make better decisions. This will also allow you to navigate and avoid potential negative speak that will put yourself in a lower vibrational state.

RULE 6: TRAVEL ABROAD

You should use every opportunity to attempt to travel and then travel even more especially out of the country. In our community we have known friends and even immediate family members that haven't even left out of their childhood neighborhoods. It could be from fear, laziness or just waiting on someone to travel with them. One of the keys to freeing yourself from the westernized matrix is to apply for and obtain a passport.

First, you will need to gather the appropriate documents and then prepare your application package. Next, you will need to find a local post office. Post offices have set hours for passport services. There you can take a passport photo and pay your passport fees. You can even check your application status online after you have submitted your application at the post office. The process is that simple.

In today's information age, there is no reason for any man to not have attempted to obtain a passport. Traveling abroad is different than just traveling stateside because you get to experience how different cultures view you as an American on a global level. I also challenge you to travel to non-westernized countries to experience another culture's way of life. It will broaden your horizons in regards to how you are treated outside the United States versus to when you are living there.

I was fortunate enough to have traveled and lived in another country during my military service which opened my eyes to how other cultures treated me with more respect than some of the people in my own country. I felt that I was treated better as a human being that demanded great respect and had value and not as an ethnicity group unlike in my own country to which I had served honorably.

While abroad I was treated as a person first and then as an American next. Because of this experience I used my passport to travel and book trips to other countries and I found that I had similar positive experiences. I strongly believe that:

"You do not truly know yourself until you have traveled alone."

Traveling alone can be an enriching, nerve wrecking and exciting experience all at the same time. When you travel alone you are forced to rely on just your street smarts and life experiences. You are truly your own man free to go and do as you wish! Traveling alone also frees you of the burden of waiting on someone else to commit to making such a decision in their life to travel with you. If you are waiting on someone to travel with you because of some perceived fears then you are just watching life past you by!

It has been said that location is everything. Sometimes by even just going to a different state out of your city people may be more responsive and positive towards you! By experiencing this welcoming attitude from other people, when you return to your local area you will start to question why people in your area aren't like that and why your area is the way that it is. That will be the catalyst for you to send a signal out to the universe to move out of that area and leave those negative people behind. While there is nothing wrong with starting to travel intermittently outside of your local area, ultimately you want to distant yourself from any place practicing a westernized culture.

While living in western culture there is a lot of propaganda about traveling outside of the country. Many people also base their ambitions to travel based on hearsay, speculations or rumors. Not facts. Many people think that once you leave the United States and travel to any country outside of it you will instantly get kidnapped and your head chopped off! This is simply untrue and not the case. These are people just trying to project their own personal fears on to you.

You may experience pushback from people in regards to traveling. They may even try to shame you from traveling at all. This is another benefit of traveling alone. Also when you travel alone to other countries you may find that more people tend to approach you than trying to approach a group or a pair of men walking together. Do you really want to have to worry about having wingmen when you are the prize in another country and the women are pursuing you? I didn't think so.

When you return from traveling abroad after having such a great time you will be less tolerant of peoples negativity in the west. It will help you to refocus on your goals of being the best version of yourself that you can be so that you can figure out the things you need to do in order to leave and travel again.

Regardless of what other people may say or think about you traveling to another country in the pursuit of happiness by following the rules in this book, you will negate the naysayers and their opinions should have zero impact on your decision making process.

You do not get points for just owning a passport. Did you know that we have foreigners living in the states that make fun of Americans that have blank passports but never use them? Take pride in being able to have stamps in your passport. You should be actively seeking to try out new cultures and experiences.

There are many benefits of traveling abroad. You improve your social and communication skills when dealing with individuals that have different traditions or customs. It also boosts your confidence. If you are able to truly move as you wish then your options in going to different places are limitless.

Traveling also creates lifetime memories that can translate to positive energy for you to put out into the universe. The endorphins that this energy creates makes you want to travel again.

Traveling helps to put your current environment in perspective to another environment that may be more favorable to your lifestyle or life choices.

Traveling also helps you to have fun and to be your truer self. You are not confined to social norms or other people's perceptions on how they feel you should think or act. When you get to travel by yourself you start to truly know yourself.

RULE 7: ESCAPING DEBTS AND EARNING NEW MONEY

Always remember, debt is slavery. We live in a consumer based economy. The United States has the largest consumer market in the entire world. Currently more than half of all millennials (classified as ages 18 to 37) will never know if or when they will be able to pay off the debts that they owe. 20% of them expect to die with some of debt. There are even systems in this country put in place that don't discharge debts after a person's death. Those debts could become the burden of their parents or even their children's responsibility. This is completely unacceptable.

Many men were born into the mindset of their parent's to go to school, graduate and then go out and get a good paying job that you will be able to use to pay your living expenses and to pay back your loans. But what happens when you have a bad economy and a lack of jobs? What do you do when the jobs readily available aren't even in your career field? What do you do about hiring discrimination and lack of spaces with ethnic hiring managers? What is being done about the exclusion of people of color as executives and in corporate settings with jobs that make real money? Men operating within westernized culture ask themselves these questions on a daily basis. Student loan debt has eclipsed all other forms of debt for the first time in 2018. That would mean that student loans debt has surpassed car loans, mortgages and credit card debt even in the aftermath of the Great Recession!

People aren't complaining or making excuses these are facts. However since we are always on our purpose the mission is to lower any existing debts as much as possible and not creating new debts until you have no debt at all. I believe that:

"Without debt you can be completely free."

Times have changed. We are about to be in the year 2020. We are living in an era where everyone is walking around with a personal computer in their pocket. There are many other ways to make money instead of just real estate or having a "job." That is the old way of making money. We want to concentrate on what could be referred to as ways of making "new money."

It is not your responsibility to convince your friends or family of how your million dollar idea is going to work. I personally have had to earn everything I ever owned. I was not privileged enough to come from a family that had generational wealth or had grandparents that passed down family businesses down to my parents then unto me. My parents did not have the money to even send me to college. I can count the amount of mentors that I had throughout my life on one finger and the one mentor that I had was when I was in my mid-thirties. It has always been just me to dig myself out of my financial situation. I don't even possess much debt just the basic necessities to operate in this system. I am sure it has been the same for a lot of men with no "safety nets."

It is extremely important that you continually read and study up on financial education and ways of making new money. Many men come from backgrounds with poor families that didn't have any sort of financial education. This information is kept hidden from average people on purpose by the 10% of the wealthy, banks and financial institutions. These institutions hold the majority of wealth. Financial education is purposely kept out of public schools. Remember this is not by coincidence. This is a system that is designed to oppress you and prevent you from making any gains to becoming the best version of yourself that you can be. It takes money to make meaningful changes in your life. Money may not make you happy but it can sure make things easier in your life! Your career and quality of life can get exponentially better because of money.

People pay individuals thousands of dollars for financial coaching and for financial advisers yet they all don't yield the same results. In matter of fact, many of them have even lost more money than they invested in learning the knowledge. While there could be many factors into why they lost that money it doesn't take a person spending that kind of money to get the knowledge required to change their financial situation.

Making new money may require you to get creative with your God given talents in order to use them to your advantage. Companies make millions of dollars off your talent doing a 9 to 5 job while underpaying you table scraps. The key is to figure out how to funnel that type of money from that company on to yourself. Your talent doesn't go away or change when you start to work for yourself so why don't you at least try to get some of that money for your own.

An example of making new money is wholesaling. The merchandise doesn't even have to be real estate anymore. It can be pretty much any product that you have access to. You can even use the internet to your advantage, a technique that we touched on in some of the subsequent rules. You can write a book or start an online business. You could become a day trader or start to invest. Those are just a few examples of making new money. Your primary use of the internet should be for obtaining the knowledge that you need to help you achieve your goals or making money. Using it for anything else is just strictly entertainment.

You may find out that many people from older generations will not understand new money or the techniques that lead to the creation of new money. They may try to shame you or pressure you into using the tactics of making old money. Some of these techniques may work while others may be obsolete. It would be wise to not discuss the specifics on how you bankroll your lifestyle with anyone.

With all new financial endeavors people may try to discourage you from your goals. There may also be jealousy towards you when you start becoming successful.

People are always pocket watching even if they don't necessarily tell you. You can make money just not more money than them. Most of this attitude comes from greedy or jealous people that lack financial education. Let your financial accomplishments speak for themselves.

RULE 8: SETTING GOALS

In order to begin any endeavor you must establish clear goals that are realistic and obtainable. These goals should have 2 classifications. They should be classified as long and short term goals. Every individual is different but you must take the time to fully flush out your goals so that you are crystal clear of the milestones that you are working towards.

Men can get easily frustrated when they are putting in the work towards their goals yet it seems that the goal remains unreachable. A person could be working towards a goal for years but not make any progress. As a result of not seeing any progress a person could give up. This is why it is important that you need to also establish obtainable short-term goals that correlate back into your main goal. By organizing your goals in this manner you can chart your progress and see how much further that you are from achieving your long-term goal.

As mentioned in Rule #3 it is important to write down your goals. Writing down and organizing your goals into short-termed goals first will help you to better organize your thoughts. That will assist you into knowing which goals have priority over the others. It will help you to know what goals to tackle first.

As you complete your tasks you should be crossing out your goals. Crossing out goals will send endorphins into your brain that will stimulate happiness, give you the energy to complete other goals and help you to relieve stress. Even while currently working a crappy 9 to 5 job that you might not enjoy just knowing that you have made time for yourself to work on your goals makes navigating through such negativity much easier.

A short-term goal is something that you want to accomplish soon. By completing these tasks in a timely manner you will start to train yourself to make goals that have a clear beginning and a clear end so that you are not idly working on tasks with no foundation or metric to measure for when that short-term goal is completed. Not establishing clear goals is a catalyst for men giving up entirely on their purpose. There is no motivation to continue because there is no light at the end of the tunnel for them to see. They are just working aimlessly through life with no direction.

A long-term goal is a goal that will be accomplished in the future. Long term goals will inspire you to do great things. Achieving long-term goals can create life altering events. Long term goals are not meant to be completed right away. These are goals that may be required to be completed further in the future after a long period of time. Wanting to be financially free in 5 years would be an example of a long-term goal.

It is also important that you don't be afraid to fail. Michael Jordan said that he failed over and over again in his life and that is why he succeeds. Failure is an opportunity to begin again, wiser and more intelligently the next time around. When you make the effort to begin again after you have failed you begin to weed out any inadequate things in your process. By doing this you will become more proficient at obtaining your goals in a timely manner. You will begin to have sure fire success because of your past experiences.

People tend to be paralyzed by the fear of failure. If you are scared of failure than you will be unable to act. When you are unable to act you are not making any progress in your life or your goals. No matter how dedicated or successful you become, your success will be determined by your ability to overcome adversity, doubt and forces that will attempt to distract or derail you from your goals. These forces could be mental, physical or economical. It is up to you to use your own will power and the techniques you have learned to ignore them.

By continually setting goals you are becoming stronger as an individual even if you are living around a negative environment. You will be conditioning yourself physically, mentally and spiritually in order to toughen yourself to any type of challenge. These actions will manifest themselves into the universe and the universe will open doors for you that wouldn't normally open if you were not on your purpose. It is not your job to figure out how the universe will open those doors. Remember the universe is neutral. Your job is just to take action.

There are reasons to why people don't reach their goals. Some people may even be intimidated or fearful of achieving their full potential. Those people may have not reached their higher purpose so they procrastinate or don't follow through on their tasks. They may also surround themselves with other people that don't reach their goals. The people that you hang around in your personal time are a reflection of the success that you have in life. Associating with people who don't have any aspirations or goals will begin to demotivate you and stifle your growth.

Sometimes a person starts too many projects but rarely follows through. These kind of actions start to cultivate a pattern of being an underachiever. An underachiever is a person who fails to achieve their greatest potential in life.

Being lazy is another catalyst of people being underachievers. There are many people living in western society that refuse to put forth the required time or effort into achieving their dreams. People such as this refuse to sacrifice anything in their personal life in order to be the best version of their selves that they could potentially be.

These types of people are happy going with the status quo and the "just going along to get along attitude" that a lot of blue pilled people have these days. Generally laziness is a lower vibration. It also can bring forth unwanted feelings such as depression, disappointment or making you feel just plain miserable. Being lazy also is a massive time waster. With that time you could be using it in to do other things that could actually benefit your situation.

You never want to settle with just being good you want to be great in all aspects of your life. Unless you hold yourself accountable for your actions and at a higher standard than the people around you then you will forever remain an underachiever. You purpose is not just come up with a bunch of goals to tackle but to actually be accomplishing them.

RULE 9: DEDICATION AND CONSISTENCY

In order for you to apply these rules into your new lifestyle you need to be consistent. Being consistent means you are dedicated to making real change in your life. When a man isn't consistent on a task it can mean that he isn't truly serious about it. By not talking things seriously or leaving tasks incomplete then those tasks become just glorified hobbies. Successful people tend to be consistent in every aspect of their life.

By practicing to be consistent it will make conquering your tasks easier overtime. Perhaps you have a goal of losing 100lbs by the end of the year. By not being consistent your weight could fluctuate up and down. The lack of not working out on days that you should be going to the gym can cause you to become unmotivated to continue the process through the very end. Even if you feel like the task isn't getting easier as long as you are consistent you are guaranteed to see results over time. In the universe consistent actions create consistent results.

Being dedicated is the act of being committed to a specific task or purpose. Most things start off as just an idea until someone is dedicated enough to manifest that idea into a reality. It takes dedication and putting in the work in order to improve yourself. It is not always going to be easy but through mental preparation and consistency you are able to overcome any task. If you learn to enjoy the process then the results will come even quicker. That is why it is so important to focus on doing the things that you like and that you want to do. It is all part of the process.

When you practice being dedicated to a task you are training yourself into being serious about taking back control of your life and becoming your true self. Serious people don't have time for things that don't add value into their lives. When people see that you are dedicated to positive things in your life other people want to be around that energy. This is how collaborations, relationships and business opportunities start.

When you are dedicated and consistent with obtaining your goals the people who may have watched you from your beginning their interactions and language towards you starts to change. They may become more inquisitive about the happenings in your life. Some may not interact with you directly but they may start taking an interest in the content you put out on your social media. While you may be mindful of how other people may interpret what you are doing, you should be consistent in doing what you are going to do regardless. You are too busy being determined to pay attention to the people that might be observing and watching you. Let your actions speak for themselves. Even if you don't get the recognition that you think you may deserve you in an outwardly manner you are not vying for anyone's confirmation or attention anyways. The cream always rises to the top.

When you are consistent and dedicated to your goals it makes it easier to accomplish them and to set new ones. When you are consistent and dedicated to the tasks in your goals it makes it quicker to accomplish one task and move to the next especially with short-term goals. Being dedicated and consistent is what separates a professional versus being a hobbyist. It shows that you are making a serious commitment and willing to put in the work in order to being the best version of yourself that you can be.

RULE 10: TAKING BACK CONTROL OF YOUR TIME

Western society is full of energy vampires who will waste and try to control your time. You need to remember time is the only commodity that you can't get back in life. People who waste your time are literally wasting your life.

Many men are working jobs that they hate. As the natural providers in society they may be in financial, economic or personal situations and feel that they cannot leave those jobs. Working a job that you do not enjoy will suck all your vitality out of you leaving you too tired to do the things that you really want to do in life. Most importantly working 40+ hours or more a week will take all your time away from yourself.

People in these types of environments all tend to share the same negative mindset. Rather they are unhappy about their pay, position, boss, or co-workers these individuals will love to try and transfer that negative energy on to you. This type of environment stifles your mental growth by locking you into situations where it creates a crabs in the barrel mentality. This type of environment is not conducive for success. You should strive to not be in any of these types of environments.

It can be argued that time is a more valuable commodity than money. You cannot get time back into your life. You should actively avoid people and tasks that are time wasters. People that do not know their purpose or have any passions may try to dictate your free time. This leaves you doing meaningless tasks that do nothing to advance your mental, physical or spiritual growth. This is very dangerous. By letting someone or some job that you do not like dictate your life you start to develop regret.

So many people living in western society have whole lives that revolve around a job that they do not enjoy doing. This job affects their personal life even when they are not at work. They may even have to make a choice between spending time with loved ones and going in to work for someone else. The majority of the management at these type of companies do not care about you as an individual, your loved ones or your passions. They are simply only using your time to advance their bottom lines and protect their quality of life. They want to ensure that they are able to enjoy their time off while you are stuck at work.

"Stop trading your time for money."

When you are dependent on someone else paying you that person may think that they are entitled to your time even when you are not at work. An example of this would be employers who like to call people constantly on their off days or have employee's working every weekend. Someone else has dictated when and when you cannot have time for yourself in your life!

This is so important why you need to develop ways of making new money as discussed in the previous rule. Ultimately you should strive to not work for anyone. You should not be dependent on someone else to pay you money. I am not saying that you have to quit your job overnight. That could be considered irresponsible especially if you have other responsibilities other than yourself. I believe that a job should only be used as a tool as advancement for succeeding at your personal goals. It should never be used to fully to dictate your quality of life or income as it could be gone at any moment.

A lot of what we have become to believe in has been passed down generationally from our parents. While these methods may have worked for them times are vastly different now. There are many ways to live a stress free life without doing a "job." People every day make money not possessing a job. Why can't you be one of those people?

Many people don't even think about the lifestyle choices that they make. They just "do." They do not take the time to think about the reasoning behind the actions that they take. A lot of it also comes from social conditioning. Society will try to force people to make choices based on a perceived notion of how it thinks a person living in its environment should behave. Society is shaped by economic trends and systems. An example of this would be the debt trap. Capitalism is the most commonly followed economic system in westernized society.

Millions of people are opting out of working for someone else and living more stress free and happier lives. These people enjoy having the ability to choose their own clients and enjoying the freedom to dictate their own time. They have the benefits of not having to ask permission to have time off to take care of their personal affairs or to just have a social life outside of working.

Many men were tricked into belief that by just working hard, getting a good education and following the law they wouldn't have any real problems and could live out their dreams. Those people quickly realize that when you live in a capitalistic society where time and wages are divided out unequally depending on your social class and ethnic group they recognize the conundrum that they are trapped into. Just having the ability to work hard is not good enough. Everyone is working hard these days. You have to take back control of your own life and you can only do that by using your time wisely and to your advantage. Do not let other people dictate your time.

Know your rights as a person and you should insist that people respect your life choices. Whenever you interact with anyone you should set boundaries from the beginning of the interaction so that people cannot just take advantage or your time. By setting boundaries you are training yourself to behave more automatically in regards to putting yourself first above other people. This ensures that people will not be able to just disregard or walk over you.

When people decide to put themselves first, other people will try to shame you by calling you selfish. Selfishness is a must for true happiness. Being selfish does not mean to be inconsiderate of others it means that you prefer to put yourself in situations where you value your time and attention in a way that puts you in the best possible situation to win at life. Selfish people have a drive to succeed and are stubborn to a point. They are not easily compelled by other people to do what those people might want them to do or be. These types of people tend to live by their own rules and walk to the beat of their own drum.

RULE 11: WORK FOR YOURSELF

If you want to build a business today we live in an era where it is the information age. You can go online and find exactly what you need to do to build any type of business. This was definitely not the case for our parents neither our grandparents. If you want freedom and to live life on your own terms then you should aspire to work for yourself.

Sometimes you need to have an honest conversation with yourself. You may feel that you are suffocating working in a 9 to 5 type of job. The job may not even see the potential in you that you see for yourself. Friends and family members may even try to tell you that stress in a work environment that stress is "normal" and that it comes with the territory. I am telling you that this is definitely not the truth nor should it be the case!

When you start to apply the rules in this book in every aspect of your life you may start to feel like that you are progressing mentally at a quicker pace than others around you or what your job may be able to provide for you. In America's rat race climate there are many men who are not progressing in their career fields due to the lack of opportunities that may be afforded to them by no fault of their own.

These jobs do not see any value in them other than being a "wage slave." A wage slave is a person that is totally financially dependent on the income of working from a 9 to 5 job. Usually while working in this type of environment if you were to lose, get fired or laid off from that job you would only be 1 or 2 weeks away from not being able to continue to pay your bills or take care of your financial responsibilities. Most states in western society have laws in place so that they can terminate employees without any proper reason or no explanation as long as they are not being discriminatory in their practices.

These companies and corporations tend to be very greedy and are very clever in using management into being discriminatory to employees without breaking any of the established state laws. Most men at these types of job are underpaid, overworked and stressed out on a daily basis. These men are often not paid a fair earning wage based on the value of their technical prowess or skills even while doing a good job for these companies. This is completely unacceptable.

You may have heard the phrase to "go out and just get a job" from close friends and family but does this type of thinking truly have your best interest at heart? The statement itself seems counterproductive with no regard to any thoughts about what you may want or your aspirations in life. Going out just to go out and get any job also disregards nontraditional or obscure careers that you may want to be involved in. These types of professionals (such as acting or game design) seem impossible to reach from people that aren't on their purpose. Remember,

"All money is not good money."

You should not do anything just for the sake of getting a paycheck. Now I am not saying that you shouldn't be beneath working something you don't necessarily like in order to make ends meet but when you should always be striving to put yourself in situations that are going to best benefit you and that you can win. Sometimes having freedom is better than money. When people become entrepreneurial and start to work for themselves people often are not going to understand what you are trying to do. You do not owe an explanation to anyone.

People often are trapped in busy schedules doing tasks that they do not care about or necessarily like. Being busy doesn't equate to working. Working for other people is a choice. Learn to not settle, you should always be striving to improve yourself. The individuals that run these companies may try to intimidate or coerce you into giving up your time for them. They feel entitled to your time just because they pay you. They want you to be dependent on their paycheck because without it you cannot make any moves. You should be increasing your business education daily. Even if you are currently working you should be working on your own personal endeavors and businesses on the side. You should be learning to make money outside this of type of system. Even getting fired means that the universe must want something better from you.

The best entrepreneurs who are successful business owners usually end up making more money on their own than if they were to be working under someone else. They also tend to regain their health, time and freedom because they were brave enough to take their own life back into their hands. If you have also been applying the rules in this book in regards to making new money you may even find that it takes less money than you think to life off of than you might be currently spending. This leaves extra money available for you to pursue even more endeavors and experiences that can better enrich your life!

When you take the leap and quit your job to work for yourself you quickly realize that you may be ill equipped and a bit lost on where to start on your journey. You start to come to the realization that if you aren't fortunate enough to come from an affluent family that society has not properly trained you on how to be entrepreneurial. The schools that you may have attended have only trained you on how to be an employee not a boss. This was by design. Because of this fact many people will make excuses on why they can't start a business. Your job is to ignore these types of people and be about your purpose.

Another important part of working for yourself you should be trying to avoid what is called performance based pay. This type of pay is usually based on labor or the amount of hours you spend while doing a task. Compensation is connected directly to how much labor that you put in. Sells would be an example of a profession that is based on performance based pay.

You should try to avoid performance based pay as much as possible and concentrate on generating passive income. Passive income is income received on consistent basis requiring minimalistic effort by the individual maintaining it. This money can grow without an individual having to tend to it at all. Receiving royalty payments would be an example of passive income. Creating an investment portfolio is a great way of generating passive income without an earner having to take an active part in generating its earnings over time. Now while passive income ideas usually require an upfront monetary investment, many of those ideas will continue to generate some form of profits or break even with little or no work to you! Passive income endeavors rarely tend to financially wipe a person out if left unchecked. You should definitely have some forms of passive income availability along with your other financial investments and endeavors.

Regardless of how other people may view or perceive you, you know your value and your worth. It is important to remember that these companies tend to need you more than you need them. Their toxic work culture is causing talented and high performing people to quit their jobs. No one wants to constantly go to a place where they feel miserable.

Many work environments consist of people that are bored and uninspired while working their jobs. When the people in charge don't have a purpose or become bored then they start to resort to negative tactics such as micromanaging, gossiping or talking down to people. This kind of culture creates a crabs in a barrel mentality.

People that start to have these kinds of traits start to develop toxic leadership habits. While they may be academically intelligent, a lot of them don't have or know the technical skills to even do the job that you were hired for! They can resort to using such tactics as giving others preferential treatment or extra privileges for people kissing their backsides. Usually this is reserved for individuals that share the same negative traits as they do.

Another common trait for people in this type of environment is that entrepreneurship is frowned upon. In today's toxic work culture the majority of people that may be in managerial types of roles did not earn the position that they were given through hard work. They were gifted these positions from families or family friends. Hiring managers even give high ranking positions to their fraternity brothers from decades ago. They will overlook more qualified applicants in spite of their ability and skills to do the job just to hire their friends or someone that they know. There is even hiring discrimination.

Because of these facts many people in management are poor leaders and they have fake interpersonal relationships with people. When your co-workers get a notion that outside of the job you may be in a better position socially than them or moving past them they may even try to sabotage your advancements. They may try to make you work longer hours than required or overtime taking away valuable time from you and for your personal aspirations and goals.

Working these types of long hours is a guaranteed way of leaving you tired and uninspired to becoming the best version of yourself that you can be. Issues at your work may even start to seep into your personal life making you more irritable towards your friends and loved ones. This type of attitude puts you in a low vibration and has a negative impact on your performance when you have time to work on goals for yourself. It is best not to mention your outside endeavors to your co-workers when you are at work or in these types of negative environments. Most of these people are not your friends. Many men in western society tend to not trust their co-workers for a variety of different reasons. You need to put your best interests first above other people.

Another common effect of just working a "job" is that men are often misplaced in positions that leave them in the wrong professional role. This leaves men working in positions that are not the right fit for them. A man may be overqualified for a position yet he is regulated to a position that is beneath is technical prowess. This person could be an exceptional leader and manager of people yet he may only be regulated to doing entry level work.

Because of this fact the person may start to underperform or seen as not good at their position. Men may even be shamed by their coworkers or punished by management for low performance. This can be detrimental to men's future career choices if they end up leaving to work for another company.

Most of companies in western society today have a revolving door policy. With the unfair At Will laws in most states these companies have no issue about letting a person go and may even hire another person for less money to replace you with. These companies do not value you as an individual or care about your livelihood. They just want a body that is dependent on the income of the job to survive.

If you are currently surviving in a toxic work culture you should be thriving to take the experience that you know at the business to be working for yourself. You should exhaust all opportunities to be in that environment as least as possible. If you have the opportunity to work from home or work part time these are options that you can use in order to funnel more time unto yourself and your goals.

RULE 12: KNOWING YOUR PURPOSE

To lead a purposeful life you must follow your passions. Your motivations drive you to find your life's purpose and influence your behavior. For some people working on their life's purpose let's people live fulfilled lives and do meaningful work. Finding your purpose directly correlates to success. In order to get what you need in life you need to know your purpose.

When you ask a person what are their passions in life people rarely have an answer. Everyone has a life purpose but most people are unconscious of it their entire lives. People will try to force your life's purpose into their perceived little boxes. Those people could be friends, family or even your managers or bosses. People like that do not see the value of you becoming your true-self and being about your purpose. They are too wrapped up in the entrapments of western culture to venture out and escape from the matrix.

Your life's purpose can be easily derailed through social, cultural, or even family conditioning. You must always be aware of these conscious and subconscious cues from other people that may put you off your path.

It is also important to remember to not have in-depth conversations with people that cannot relate to your struggles. The majority of the time these types of conversations can become argumentative or the person will not understand your ambitions or goals. It is not for them to understand! You only have one life and your purpose is for you and you alone. Only you will know what your life's purpose is.

You should commit to expressing yourself in the way that you would want to live your life's purpose. If you might want to be in the entertainment industry as a prominent figure there is nothing wrong with carrying yourself in the way you would like to be portrayed or seen. You may receive some pushback from individuals but remember that by doing this you are already externalizing your life's purpose onto yourself and the universe.

Not everyone will be a risk taker such as yourself just in the same way not everyone joins the military. For example some people view joining the military in a positive way while some people view it as a negative. When you externalize your purpose you are doing the same thing. Some people may support your new endeavors while others may hate on you. As mentioned in Rule #8 if you already have clear cut goals established you are going to be too busy to notice the noise around you regardless.

You will need to try to reestablish self-confidence and lost self-esteem from spending so much time in a negative environment. As mentioned in Rule #6 traveling abroad may assist you in manifesting your goal into reality. Maybe it might take you externalizing your life's purpose in a different environment in order for you to get into the groove of your new role and purpose in life. Do not let the negativity and noise in your current situation and environment bring you down!

Your life's purpose cannot be too big nor too small. You have to remember that regardless of the perils you may face in everyday life your options are limitless. The most important thing is to find out what will drive you and energize you to move forward with your purpose.

This may takes some self-introspection. You need to be true to yourself and internalize your inner feelings to ask the pertinent questions of yourself. What makes you happy? What do you want out of life? What do you love to do? What are you willing to sacrifice to reach your goals?

We live in a society where it is frown upon for people to ask questions. Our bosses and managers do not like to be questioned. Even our educators don't like to be questioned! In today's culture everyone is scared to say anything that goes against society's norms. Yet people will allow someone else to put their own livelihoods in peril because they are too afraid to ask the right questions.

Notice that I mentioned the "right" questions. If you were drowning you wouldn't ask when will the mailman arrive, you would ask when is help going to arrive to save you! The questions you ask should always be pertinent based on the situation that is presented in front of you at the time.

Knowing your purpose also influences your behavior. When you are working on your purpose you are giving out positive signals to the universe. The universe naturally responds by opening doors for you that will help you achieve your goals. When you are giving positive signals to the universe you are in the state of creating high vibrations. When you are in that vibrational state the universe gives you energy and your body absorbs that energy and it motivates you to put in the work towards your goals. When your high vibrations past their natural thresholds that is when you start to achieve amazing things! That is when long term goals get completed.

RULE 13: BE SOLUTION-ORIENTED

Being solution-oriented means as a man you should be changing your attitude in regards to figuring out solutions to any situation in your life. It is vastly important to remember that to have solutions means that you are giving yourself options. We must discipline ourselves to adopt a winner mindset. People that constantly give reasons on why a problem exists or can't be figured out are complainers. Being around these types of people do not cultivate an environment for success. Being solution-oriented means that you are channeling energy not to stand paralyzed in the face of a problem.

We must employ creative methods sometimes in order to find solutions to a problem. You may encounter people that will present problems and complain but do not ever come up with a solution to the problem. Some of these people are chronic complainers. These people don't even want to attempt to solve problems even if they are given clear solutions to those problems. They just want to complain for the sake of complaining. You should avoid people with this character trait at all cost.

By allowing someone like this into your space when you are problem solving the environment tends to become polluted with negativity and it lowers everyone's vibrations that person has contact with. Even in toxic environments people don't like to be around people who complain all the time.

By shifting your attitude and mindset into becoming more solution-oriented it helps you to break through the barriers of finding an actual solution to your problem. It also allows you to see all the possible outcomes when searching for an answer to your problem. A good technique is not to say "I can't" rather to say "how can I?" By simply changing your attitude it changes your entire approach to the problem!

By being solution-oriented you will start to think more methodical and strategically which will help you to make more informed and better decisions. By taking the time to find all the possible outcomes to the problem you are presented with then you are in a better position to have a contingency plan for all the possible outcomes. This makes you truly prepared and not just relying on luck or time to solve your problems. You are taking a proactive approach to moving forward and not dwelling on what perceived notions on what you can't do.

Being solution-oriented also allows you to look at situations for what they are. Those situations could be positive or negative. Do not get emotionally involved with the problem. Tackle the problems with your focus and dedication in order to move past them.

When you are solution-oriented you are training yourself to actually becoming more intelligent and clever in the methodology of how you move in life. You tend to be more focused on resolving challenged based tasks than avoiding them. You also tend to be more focused on accomplishment and seeing problems completely through to their end. This decreases the chances of you not completing goals that you have set for yourself. You have identified yourself as not allowing limitations to dictate what you can and cannot do in life. You should strive to be limitless in every aspect of your life. Being limitless gives you the ability to open opportunities and have options in your life.

CONCLUSION:

Living in western society can be a stressful and challenging endeavor but by using the techniques mentioned in this book you will have the ability to confront any challenge with the confidence and positivity you will need to accomplish your goals.

You will start to notice that in your personal life a multitude of distractions have increasingly taken over your ability from achieving everything that you wanted to do in your life. You will be able to differentiate those distractions into distinct categories, those that are just means to an end with a clear end goal or distractions that are overtaking your life to the point that you are unhappy and unable to act. Rather these distractions exist in your personal or professional life, you will be able to see those distractions as to what they truly are and you will be motivated to do what you will need to do in order to overcome them and to be the best version of yourself that you want to be.

To be successful in life you will realize that a person must value their time and that your time is very important. No one can regain time that is lost. You will be less tolerant of people or activities that waste your time and that prevent you from achieving your goals.

You will start to identify people that do not add value to your life and as you succeed in spite of those types of people you will leave some people in your life behind. Through your success the universe will provide to you people to replace the ones lost and those people will share common interests. Those people will start to enrich your life and you will enrich the lives of others.

You will be productive and effective and you will live a much more fulfilling and healthy life by traveling abroad. You will become a more knowledgeable and well-rounded individual by experiencing new cultures and economic norms outside of the western matrix.

You will be able to generate new money outside of current economic systems and that money will allow you to pay off the debts from old money and generate additional streams of income. That money will allow you to reinvest into yourself and your ambitions.

Most importantly, you will know what your purpose is in life will be and you will be able to set goals for yourself that you will overcome by using dedication and consistency.

www.ingramcontent.com/pod-product-compliance
Lightning Source LLC
Chambersburg PA
CBHW061739250726

48657CB00002B/1002